EASY KETO DESSERTS

By

Lyndi Kae

Decadent Deserts

excerpts, you may contact the author at lyndi-kae.author@gmail.com. This book is licensed for your personal enjoyment only. An eBook may not be sold or given away to other people. If you would like to share the book, please do so through proper retail channels. If you are reading the eBook and did not purchase it or it was not purchased for you, please return it and purchase your own copy. Please respect the legal rights and hard work of the author. Characters and some locations in this book are fictional and figments of the author's imagination. Characters, locations or events portrayed _ctionally associating or interacting with _ctional characters in the story are portrayed in ways feasible; however, their experiences are _ctional and of the author's imagination. Any similarity of _ctional characters or events in this book to actual characters and events is purely conjecture on the part of the author, for the sake of entertainment only. The author is not a dietitian, medical practitioner or nutritionist. No medical or legal claims are made by this book. It is meant to be a tool useful to the reader and nothing more. As with any diet, consult your physician before beginning the program.

Email: lyndikae.author@gmail.com
Website: https://for-yous.com/
Or
http://www.lyndareesauthor.com
Facebook: @ForYouABetterLife

As with any diet program, it is recommended you consult your doctor before beginning.

Easy Keto Desserts

Decadent Desserts
By
Lyndi Kae

Email: lyndikae.author@gmail.com Website:https://
HOW-TO-KETO.COM
Website: https://for-yous.com/
Also https://lyndareesauthor.com
Original Edition
Copyright © 2020
Publisher: Sweetwater Publishing Company
6694 Ky. Hwy. 17 North
DeMossville, KY 41033

Table of Contents

Overview

Introduction

Chapter 1, Breads

- Soft Taco Shells
- Cloud Bread
- Low Carb Bread
- Fried Bread
- Pizza Crust
- Quick Bread
- Bread of Life
- Keto Biscuits
- Keto Crepes

Chapter 2, Decadent Desserts

- Sweet Snack
- Pumpkin Pie
- Dark Chocolate Cherry Bites
- Chocolate Cake Cup
- Somoa Cookies
- Berry Quinoa Bites
- Pumpkin Cookies
- Berry Creamy Delight
- Chocolate Pudding
- Whipped Topping
- Individual Birthday Cake
- Creamy Cake Frosting
- Berry Popsicles
- Chocolate Strawberries
- Chocolate Chip Bars
- Meringue
- Mousse 'Cupcakes'
- Ice Cream
- Chocolate Fudge

Chapter 8, Yummy Drinks

- Keto Friendly Drinks
- Chocolate Milk Shake
- Berry Spritzer

Also By Lyndi Kae

OVERVIEW

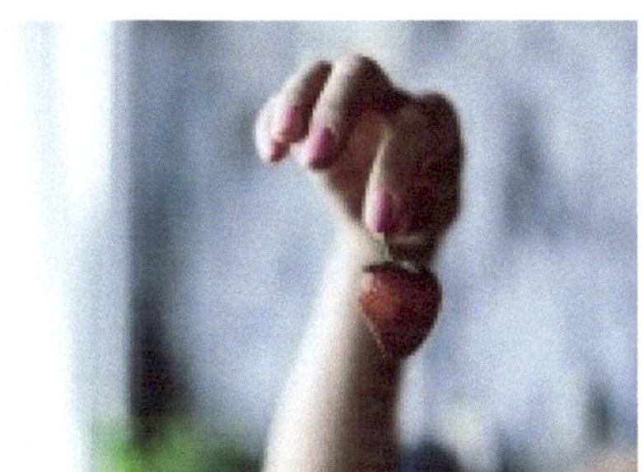

This cookbook is a tool to help you start and stick to your Ketogenic Diet. This life changing eating process shouldn't be difficult.

The book is written to make your life easier and to help the ketogenic lifestyle become second nature. These delectable recipes will help you not only stick to your Keto Diet. They will help you relish and enjoy it.

These fabulous recipes are filled with antioxidants and healthy fats to improve focus and help you feeling free and amazing.

Just because you're on an eating plan to lose weight and maintain a healthy lifestyle, doesn't mean you must skip dessert. Heck no!

This book provides recipes for delectable breads, decadent dessert and delightful drinks so rich you won't be deprived in the least. In fact, you'll feel pampered—maybe even downright sinful.

INTRODUCTION

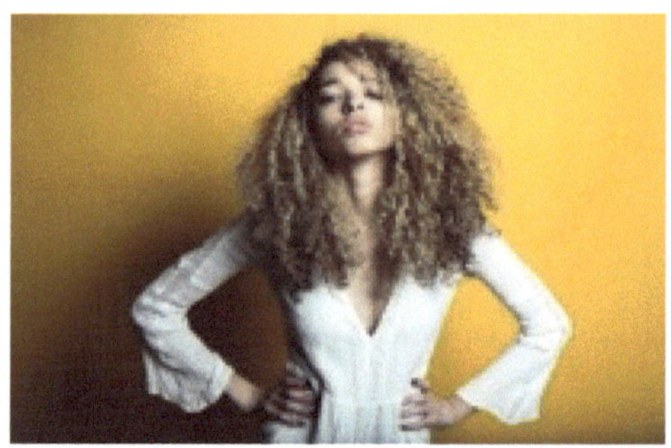

Whether you're an experienced Keto Dieter looking for fun recipes or a newbie trying to satisfy your sweet tooth, you've come to the right place.

This book is for you.

These delights are designed to promote your Ketogenic Dieting efforts and Keto Diet strategies for weight loss and health improvement.

No counting calories—just enjoy these simple, quick-to-prepare recipes that allow you to stay in ketosis so you shed weight.

As with any program, the Keto Diet only works if you are consistent and stick to it. So these good fat, medium protein and low carb desserts will satisfy your craving for sweets and help you attain your goal.

There is no special market to seek out. No exotic foods you must find to prepare Decadent Keto Desserts. Everything you need is readily accessible wherever you normally shop.

You're going to love these delectable recipes.

Jump in. Let's eat!

CHAPTER 1
Breads

Most people don't think of bread as a dessert. Your body absorbs regular, wheat-based bread starches and convert them into sugar to be burned by your body for fuel. On a KETO Diet you avoid those starchy breads, so your body burns fat for fuel.

Many consider bread comfort food. Some KETO dieters crave bread or miss convenience of including bread to prepare sandwiches or to accompany certain dishes. If you're one of those bread-craving folks, you're going to appreciate these simple bread recipes.

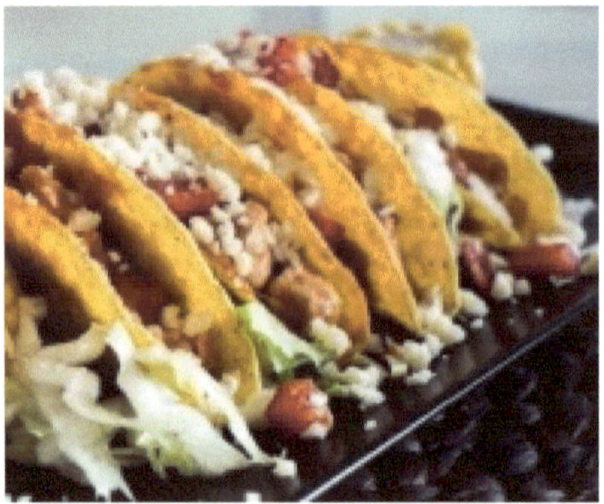

Soft Taco Shells

Cooking time: 10 minutes
Ingredients:

Pinch salt
1 Egg
1 Cup water
1 Cup almond or coconut flour
1 Teaspoon baking powder
1 Teaspoon xanthan gum
Butter for frying.

Instructions:

Mix ingredients and make small balls. Place on waxed paper. Flatten with a rolling pen until size you want. Refrigerate to set. Heat butter in skillet. Fry gently until lightly brown on each side. Enjoy with lots of meat, real sour cream, peppers, lettuce, tomatoes and real cheese. Skip the beans, as they're high in carbs.

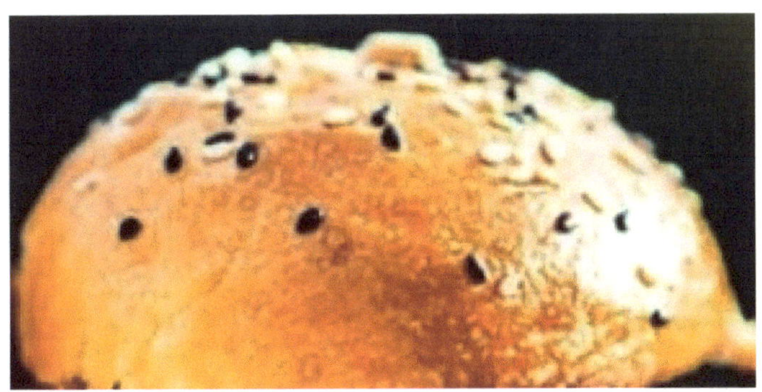

Cloud Bread

Cooking time: 15 minutes
Ingredients:

1 Cup mozzarella cheese
¼ Cup almond flour
1 Egg
1 Teaspoon garlic bread
Butter for pan.

Instructions:

Heat oven 350 degrees. Grease pan. Mix ingredients and place in prepared pan. Bake 15 minutes.

Low Carb Bread

Cooking time: 50 minutes
Ingredients:

1 Tablespoon scallions
1 Tablespoon herb of choice (oregano, parsley, etc.)
1 Large egg
1 Tablespoon olive oil
1 Tablespoon almond flour
¼ Teaspoon baking powder
1 Tablespoon coconut flour
Pinch salt
¼ Cup grated cheddar cheese
1 Tablespoon milk
2 Tablespoons butter or bacon grease for pan

Instructions:

Preheat oven to 400 degrees. Grease bread pan with butter or bacon grease. Mix remaining ingredients and make place in prepared bread pan. Bake 30-45 minutes until the center is done and crust is to the desired golden color.

Fried Bread

Cooking time: 10 minutes
Ingredients:

1 Egg
1 ½ Cup mozzarella, shredded
¾ Cup almond flour
¼ Cup bacon grease

Instructions:

Heat bacon grease in skillet on medium. Mix remaining ingredients and make patties. Place in heated grease. Fry each side about 2 minutes per side, or until desired shade of gold. Continue until the whole batch is done. Yum!

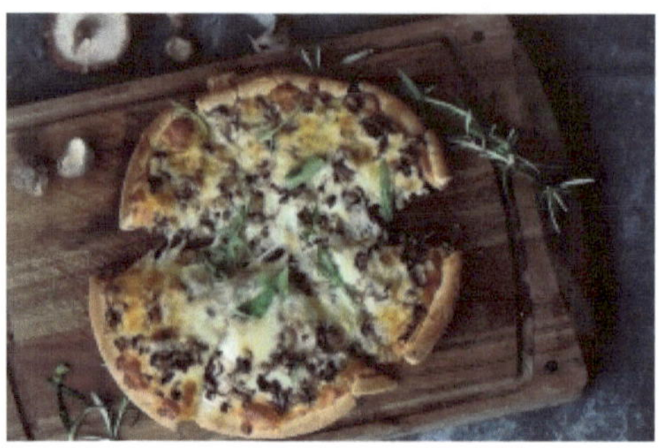

Pizza Crust

Cooking time: 25 minutes

Ingredients:

1 Cup coconut flour
7 Eggs
½ Teaspoon baking powder
Salt & pepper to taste
1 Tablespoon garlic powder
1 Dash cayenne
1 Tablespoon Italian spices
2 Tablespoons olive oil

Instructions:

Preheat oven to 375 degrees. Whisk eggs. Mix remaining ingredients until well combined into a dough ball. Press into a small pizza pan. Brush with olive oil. Bake 20-25 minutes until lightly brown. Cool. Top with keto friendly sauce and approved toppings of choice.

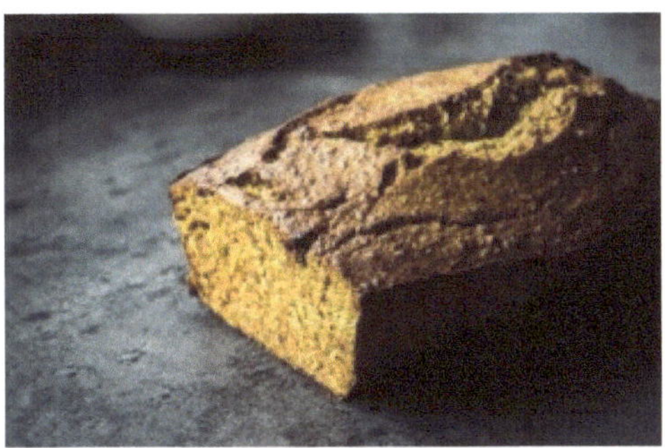

Quick Bread

Cooking time: 10 minutes
Ingredients:

½ Cup almond flour
2 Tablespoons coconut flour
2 Eggs
1 Teaspoon baking powder
1 Teaspoon cayenne
Dash salt
2 Tablespoons coconut oil, melted
2 Teaspoon garlic powder
2 Tablespoons butter for pan

Instructions:

Heat oven to 350 degrees. Grease a bread or cake pan with butter. Mix ingredients. Pour into greased pan. Bake 8-10 minutes in cake pan to golden brown, slightly longer in bread pan. Serve slices warm.

Bread of Life

I call this bread of life because it is fabulous and makes you feel decadent while doing something great for your body. I'm a bread lover—breads of all kinds.

NOTE: For variation, add more garlic. You can also add paprika, cumin, or even taco seasoning for a variety of flaors.

Cooking time: 10 minutes
Ingredients:

6 Eggs
1 1/2 Cup almond flour
1 Tablespoon baking powder
1 Teaspoon cream of tartar
Dash salt
Dash of garlic powder
Oil for pan

Instructions:

Heat oven to 350 degrees. Grease bread pan with oil. Mix eggs and spices in a bowl. Mix flour and baking powder in another bowl. Mix wet ingredients into dry ones until this forms a batter. Put into prepared pan. Spray the top with oil. Bake approximately 10 minutes until golden.

Keto Biscuits

Cooking time: 10 minutes
Ingredients:
   ½ Teaspoon chili powder
   ½ Teaspoon baking powder
   1 Teaspoon garlic powder
   Salt and black pepper to taste
   2 Eggs
   4 Tablespoons butter
   1 Cup cheddar cheese
   3 Oz. cream cheese
   1 Cup almond flour
   ½ Cup sour cream or whole fat yogurt

Instructions:

Heat oven to 425 degrees F. Soften butter, cream and cheddar cheeses. Mix with sour cream or yogurt and eggs. Add spices and baking powder. Add almond flour and make into a dough ball. Pull in half, then half the two balls, continue breaking balls apart until you have biscuit sized balls. Place on greased baking sheet. Bake 8-12 minutes, until they have risen and are golden brown. Serve hot with butter.

Keto Crepes

This decadent dessert looks fancy and is sure to impress your guest. Fact is, it's simple and a breeze to prepare.

Cooking time: 5 minutes
Ingredients:
¾ Cup almond flour
3 Eggs
1 Tablespoon approved sweetener or stevia
2 Tablespoons heavy whipping cream
2 Oz. cream cheese, softened
1 Teaspoon cinnamon
1 Teaspoon nutmeg
1 Teaspoon vanilla
Butter
3 Oz. cream cheese, softened
2 Teaspoons Splenda or powdered Splenda
1 Teaspoon vanilla or flavouring of choice
1 Teaspoon cocoa or melted dark chocolate (optional)
1 Cup mixed berries (or berry of choice)

Instructions:

Heat a skillet on medium burner. Melt butter in skillet. Whip cream until frothy. Whip in soften cream cheese and vanilla. Mix dry ingredients in a separate bowl. Add dry ingredients to whipped mixture and blend until smooth. If not thin enough, add another tablespoon of cream. Spoon desired sized portions into skillet. Cook on medium heat until the center starts to bubble, about 1-2 minutes. Flip and cook remaining size about 1-2 minutes, until it's the desired shade of brown. Remove to plate to cool. Repeat until batch is done. Fill with cream mixture and berries.

Cream mixture: In separate bowl, combine 3 oz. softened cream cheese, vanilla, cocoa (if you choose) and sweetener. Whip to soft. Fold in berries. Divide mixture among crepes. Roll each to hold filling.

Serve hot. This can be topped with chocolate chips, berries or all-fruit preserves. Check carb count on label of preserves.

CHAPTER 2
Sweeteners

As you create these desserts, be sure to use natural sweeteners that won't take you out of Ketosis. There are several safe substitutes. Feel free to experiment with them and determine which one is your favorite to use in these recipes.

On a low-carb diet or KETO Diet, you should avoid sugar, honey, maple syrup and other forms of sugar, which are high in carbs but low in nutrients. Raw honey is a natural sweetener filled with nutrients and has been shown to slow sugar absorption in the intestines to cut risk of blood glucose spikes by 50%, according to the Journal of Medicinal Food. However, it may **not** be the sweetener for you on this diet plan. Carbs in honey may take you over your daily allotment to stay in Ketosis. There are approximately 17 grams carbohydrates per 1 tablespoon of honey.

I personally prefer Splenda for most of my cooking. Splenda Zero® Liquid Sweeteners have no calories or carbohydrates, so they can be used freely without concern for carbohydrate counting. Powdered Splenda can be substituted for sugar in a one-to-one ratio for most recipes. Use to sweeten drinks or foods not requiring high temperature cooking. You may want to stick to other sweeteners for baking. Splenda contains dextrose and maltodextrin, which could possibly kick you out of ketosis. If you find this to be true in your case, look for other optional sweeteners.

Powdered stevia is a great option derived from a plant. It's considered a non-nutritive, natural sweetener and contains little-to-no calories or carbs. Unlike sugar, animal and human studies have shown stevia may help lower blood sugar levels.

Monk fruit is another splendid option for a sweetener. Never heard of monk fruit? This no sugar choice doesn't affect blood sugar levels, has no carbs, no calories and is deemed safe by the U. S. Food and Drug Administration. Monk fruit is sold at most retailers and readily available on the internet.

Whatever you use, be conscious of carbohydrate content. Check labels to be sure you stay within your daily carb allotment, so you will stay in fat burning ketosis.

CHAPTER 3
Decadent Desserts

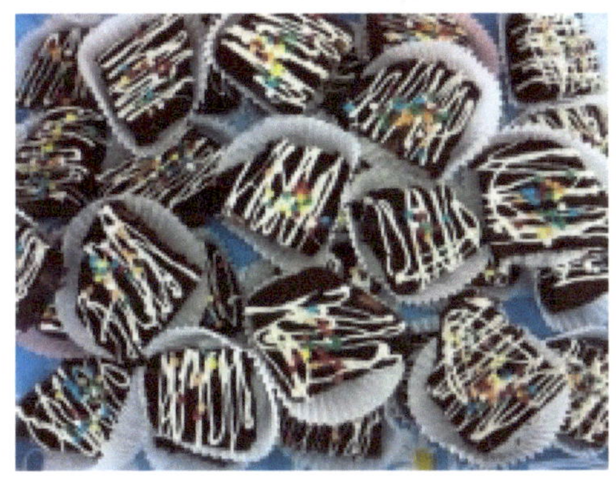

Quinoa Fruit Salad

Quinoa is a grain but is extremely high in protein. It provides a great alternative to noodles, potatoes or other starches in meals. It's delicious cooked by itself for breakfast, lunch or dinner as a side dish, or combined with other ingredients in many recipes. This delightful addition to any salad or wrap, can be used as a side dish with or without adding your preferred spices.

Quinoa is a wonderful way to add protein and bulk to a enchanting fruit salad.

Cooking time: 5 minutes
Ingredients:

- 1 Box quinoa cooked as recommended
- 2 Cups greens
- 1 Medium chopped apple
- 1 Chopped stalk of celery (optional)
- ¼ Cup raisins
- ¼ Cup dried cranberries
- ¼ Cup nuts
- 2 Tablespoons sesame seeds
- 2 Cups mixed berries or berry of choice
- 1 Tablespoon lemon juice
- 1 Tablespoon wine vinegar
- 1 Tablespoon olive oil
- 2 Tablespoons heavy whipping cream
- ½ Teaspoon MCT oil
- 1 Tablespoon Splenda or powdered stevia

Instructions:

Dressing: In small bowl, combine cream, sweetener, vinegar, juice, sesame seeds, MCT and olive oil. Eliminate cream, if you prefer a clear dressing.

Mix other ingredients in larger bowl. Pour dressing over. Toss.

Serve immediately. If prepared ahead of time, refrigerate and wait until ready to serve to add dressing.

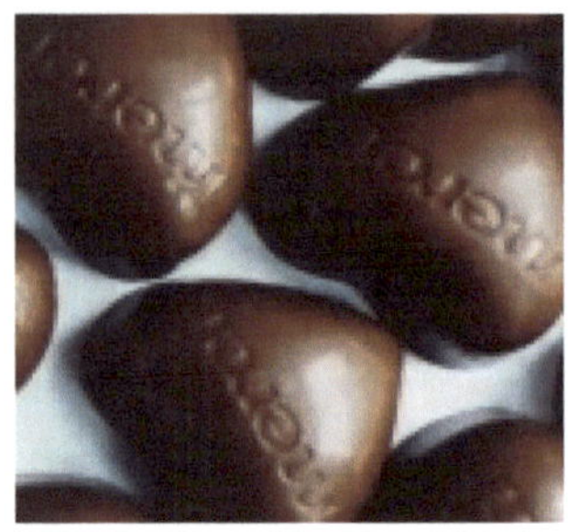

Sweet Snack

Cooking time: 0 minutes
Preparation time: 5 minutes
Ingredients:

1 Cup melted dark chocolate
1 Avacado, deseeded and peeled.
1 Tablespoon melted coconut oil
1 Teaspoon vanilla
½ Teaspoon salt

Instructions:

Mix ingredients and make balls. Place on waxed paper. Refrigerate to set. Enjoy.

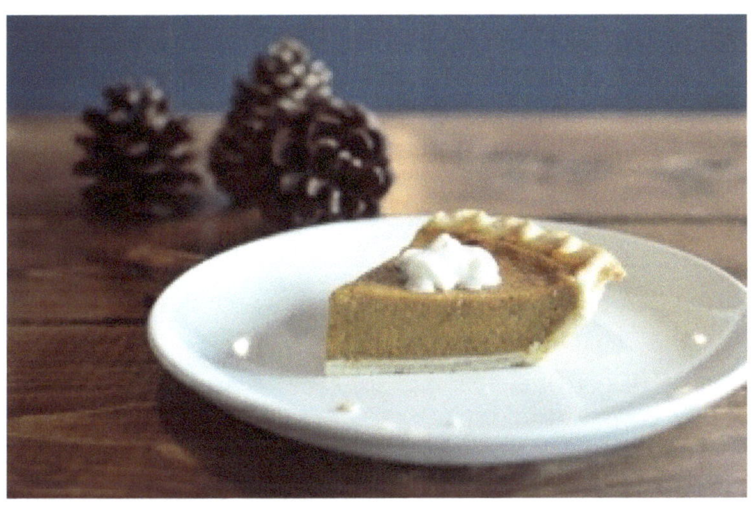

Pumpkin Pie

Cooking time: 60 minutes

Ingredients:

Crust:
   2 Cups almond flour
   1 Teaspoon cinnamon
   1 Teaspoon nutmeg or pumpkin pie spice
   1 Egg yolk
   1 Teaspoon vanilla
   1 Tablespoon Splenda or stevia
   4 Tablespoon melted butter
   1 Teaspoon coconut oil

Instructions:

Heat oven to 400 degrees. Mix ingredients and press into a pie pan greased with coconut oil. Bake 10-12 minutes until golden.

Filling:
  3 Large eggs
  1 Egg white
  1 Tablespoon vanilla
  2 Tablespoons pumpkin pie spice
  8 Oz. cream cheese, softened
  Dash salt
  1 Small can pumpkin puree (not pumpkin filling)
  1 Cup whipping cream
  ¾ Cup Splenda or powdered stevia

Instructions:

Whip eggs, cream, vanilla, sweetener and spices until you achieve a heavy froth. Add remaining ingredients and fold until combined. Pour into baked shell. Bake 45 minutes, or until done in middle. Cool 15 minutes. Serve. Keep refrigerated.

This pie is delicious when topped with Whipped Topping. Recipe can be found later in this section.

Dark Chocolate Cherry Bites

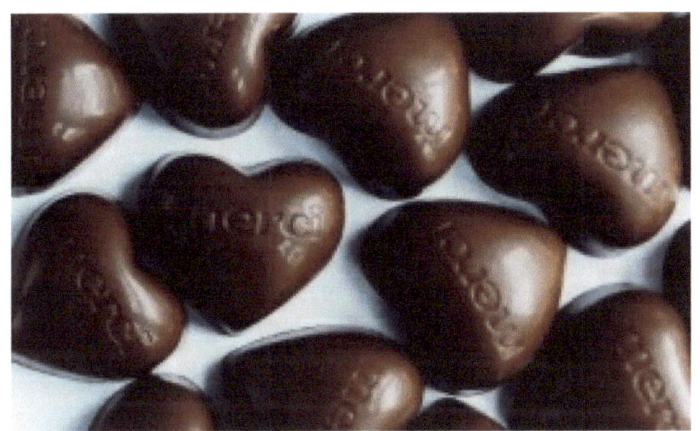

Preparation time: 5 minutes
Ingredients:

- 1 Cup pitted cherries, fresh
- 10 Pitted dates
- 2 Cups chopped almonds, raw
- ¼ Cup mini dark chocolate chips
- Pinch salt
- 2 Teaspoons water

Instructions:

Mix ingredients and make balls. These no-bake goodies are sure to delight your whole family.

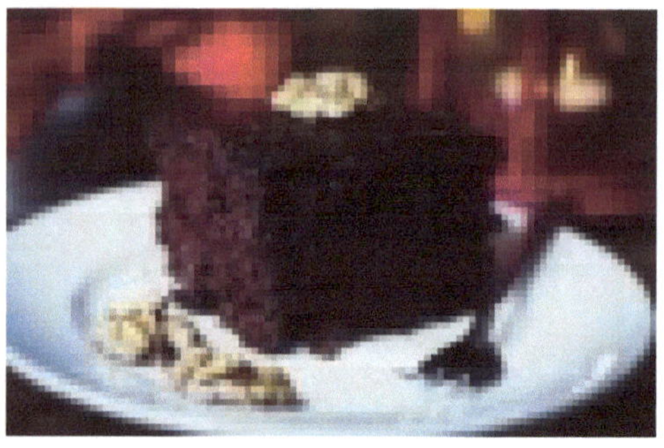

Chocolate Cake Cup

Cooking time: 6 minutes

Ingredients:

3 Oz. soften creamed cheese
½ Teaspoon stevia
¼ Cup almond flour
¼ Cup coconut flour
¼ Cup cocoa
Dash salt
1 Teaspoon baking powder
1 Large egg
¼ Teaspoon vanilla
Coconut oil or butter to grease cup
2 Tablespoons melted dark chocolate (optional)

Instructions:

Mix dry ingredients in a small bowl. Grease cup. Mix egg and whipping cream in cup with a fork. Add cream cheese and vanilla. Blend. Add dry ingredients and mix to combine. Bake in microwave approximately 1.5 minutes until done. Eat from the cup or turn upside down on serving dish. Rap sides to loosen and tap bottom to release. Drizzle dark chocolate over and serve warm or cool. Optional, decorate with chopped nuts. If you choose to ice the cake, let it cool completely first. Ice it gently. The cake will be delicate.

Samoa Cookies

Preparation time: 5 minutes
Ingredients:

1 Cup fresh coconut
1 Cup pitted, chopped dates
½ Teaspoon coconut oil
Dash salt
1 Teaspoon vanilla
1/3 Cup dark chocolate

Instructions:

Mix ingredients except for chocolate. Ball them. Lay on waxed paper. Flatten balls. Punch a hole in the center of each. Refrigerate to set. Melt chocolate. Drizzle over cookies in stripes. Refrigerate to set chocolate.

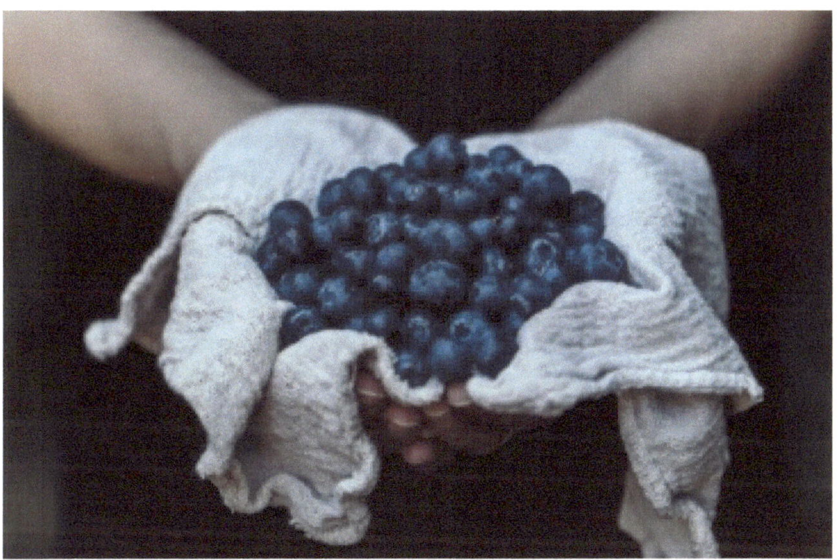

Berry Quinoa Bites

Preparation time: 5 minutes
Ingredients:

1 Box quinoa, prepared as directed and cooled.
1 Cup any variety of berries you prefer
½ Cup almond flour
½ Cup chopped nuts of your preference

Instructions:

Mix ingredients and make balls. Place on waxed paper. Refrigerate to set. Enjoy.

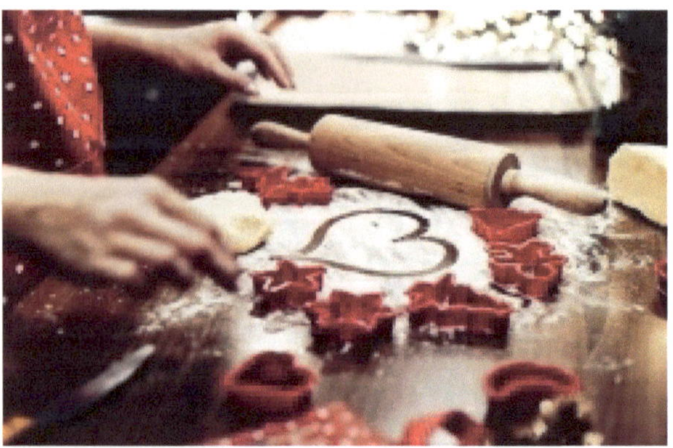

Pumpkin Cookies

Cooking time: 10 minutes
Ingredients:

1 Cup pumpkin puree, not pumpkin pie filling
1 Teaspoon baking soda
¼ Cup almond flour
½ Teaspoon vanilla
¼ Cup almond flour
2 Tablespoons honey
Butter to grease pan

Instructions:

Heat oven to 350 degrees. Mix ingredients. Use ice cream dipper to scoop cookies onto prepared baking sheet. Bake 8-12 minutes until set. Cool. Enjoy these delightful treats.

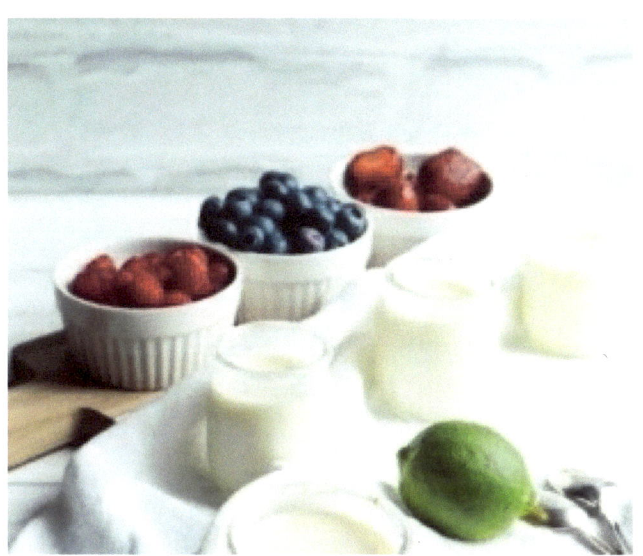

Berry Creamy Delight

Preparation time: 2 hours 15 minutes
Ingredients:

- 2 Cups strawberries or berry of choice
- 1 Cup powdered stevia
- 16 Oz. heavy whipping cream
- 1 Teaspoon vanilla

Instructions:

In a bowl, mash berries to a pulp. Add sweetener and vanilla then mix. Cool 10 minutes. In a separate cold, metal bowl, whip heavy cream until peaks form. Fold in berry mixture. Put into dessert dishes. Refrigerate for 2-3 hours. Serve.

Chocolate Pudding

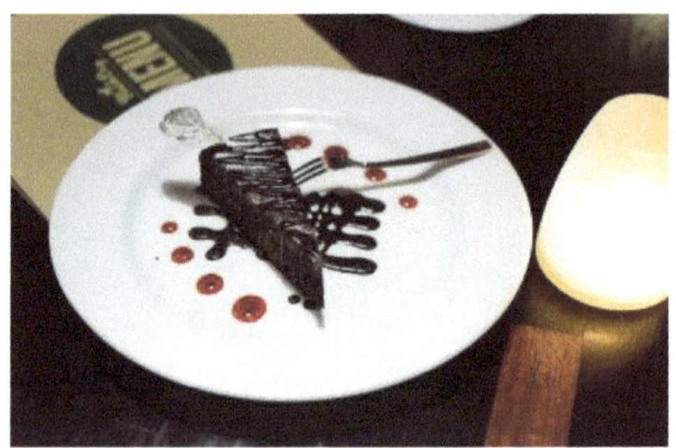

Preparation time: 65 minutes
Ingredients:

- 2 Pureed avocados
- 3 Tablespoons honey
- 1 Teaspoon vanilla
- ½ Cup cocoa powder

Instructions:

Mix ingredients. Cover and chill for an hour. This pudding is awesome with whipped topping atop it.

Whipped Topping

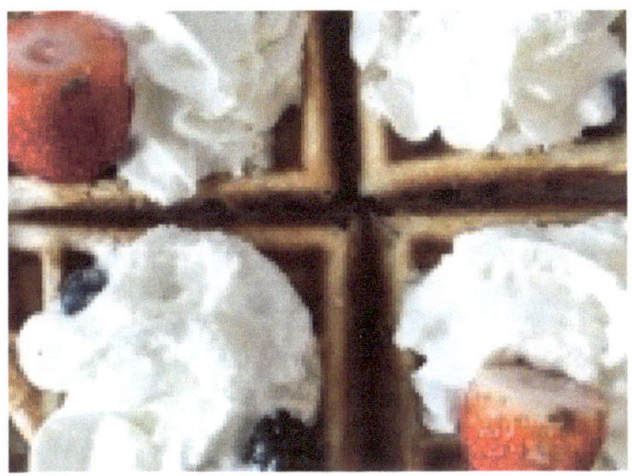

Preparation time: 10 minutes
Ingredients:

- 1 Cup heavy whipping cream
- 1 Teaspoon vanilla
- 1 Teaspoon cream of tartar
- 2 Teaspoons powdered stevia

Instructions:

Chill your mixer's whisks. Mix ingredients. Using chilled mixer whisks, whip on high speed until firm peaks appear. Keep chilled.

Individual Birthday Cake

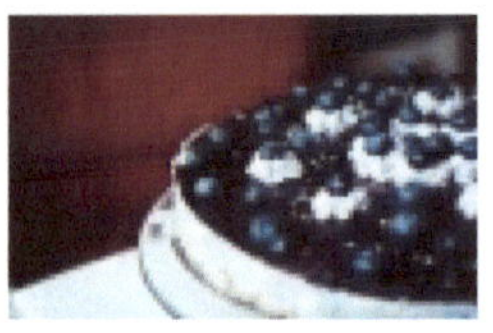

Cooking time: 6 minutes
Ingredients:

3 Oz. soften creamed cheese
½ Teaspoon Splenda or powdered stevia
¼ Cup almond flour
¼ Cup coconut flour
Dash salt
1 Teaspoon baking powder
1 Large egg
2 Tablespoons heavy whipping cream
½ Teaspoon vanilla
Coconut oil or butter to grease cup

Instructions:

Mix dry ingredients in a small bowl. Grease cup. Mix egg, vanilla and whipping cream in cup with a fork. Add cream cheese and whip. Add dry ingredients and mix to combine. Bake in microwave approximately 1.5 minutes, until done. Turn cup upside down on serving dish. Rap sides of cup slightly to loosen and tap bottom to release cake. Cool completely. Ice carefully, as cake will be delicate.

Creamy Cake Frosting

Cooking time: 6 minutes
Ingredients:

2 Oz. soften creamed cheese
2 Tablespoons Splenda or powdered stevia
1 Tablespoon softened unsalted butter
1 Tablespoon heavy whipping cream
½ Teaspoon vanilla
Food coloring, optional

Instructions:

Chill beaters and metal bowl. Whip cream, sweetener and vanilla until it peaks. Whip in soft butter and soft cream cheese. If you want to decorate with colored frosting, divide needed amounts into small bowls. Using a fork, mix in a drop or two of each color in each bowl. Carefully decorate cake, as icing may stick firmly and Keto cakes tend to be soft and delicate. You're ready to celebrate!

Variation: For chocolate frosting, add 1/4 cup cocoa or 2 oz. melted dark bakers chocolate as you blend cream cheese into frosting.

Berry Popsicles

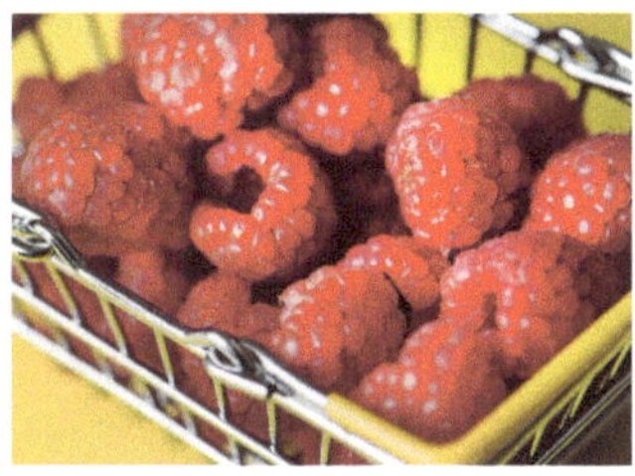

Preparation time: 10 minutes
Ingredients:

1 Cup berries, any variety or combination
½ Cup powdered stevia
½ Teaspoon vanilla
1 Cup heavy whipping cream
Popsicle sticks and molds or small cups

Instructions:

In a bowl, mix berries with stevia. Cool for 15 minutes. Add vanilla and blend berries to smooth. In a separate cold, metal bowl, whipping cream to firm. Fold berry mixture in. Pour into molds and insert sticks. Put into freezer for 4-6 hours. When ready to enjoy, simply run mold under water and squeeze to release. Enjoy this delightful way to cool off on a hot, summer day.

Chocolate Strawberries

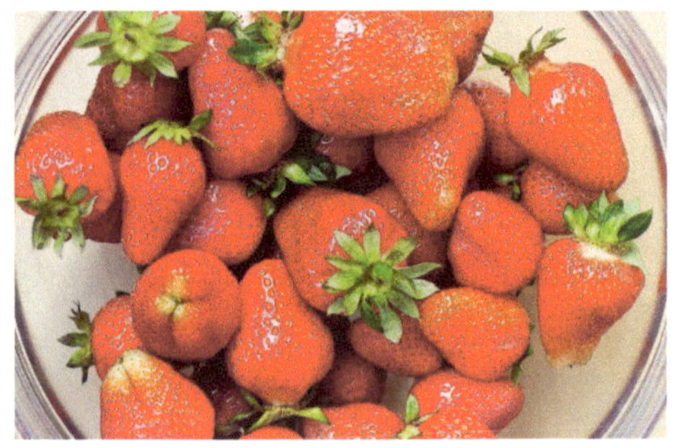

Preparation time: 10 minutes
Ingredients:

1 Pint fresh strawberries
¼ Cup dark chocolate

Instructions:

Wash and dry berries. In a small bowl melt dark chocolate in microwave. Suggest stirring every 30 seconds so you don't burn it. Holding stem side, dip berries so they emerge halfway into chocolate. Lift. Place them on wax paper to dry or into individual cupcake liners. Speed drying time by refrigerating coated berries a few minutes. They're ready to serve. Enjoy this decadent treat. Present it as an elegant gift to a loved one in a fancy box or dish, or take it to your next get together to wow your friends.

Chocolate Chip Bars

Preparation time: 2 hours
Ingredients:

1 Cup vanilla almond milk
1 Teaspoon almond flavouring
4 Tablespoons melted coconut oil
¾ Cup Non-carb vanilla protein powder
1 Tablespoon vanilla extract
¼ Teaspoon salt
3 Tablespoon Splenda or powdered stevia
2 Oz. Chocolate chips

Instructions:

Line 9"x9" pan with parchment paper. In bowl, mix dry ingredients. Mix wet ingredients in a cup. Pour mixed wet ingredients into dry ones. Blend by hand with spoon. Pour into baking pan. Cover with parchment paper. Press down on paper to compress. Refrigerate 2-4 hours. Cut into bars or squares. Enjoy! Store sealed in refrigerator.

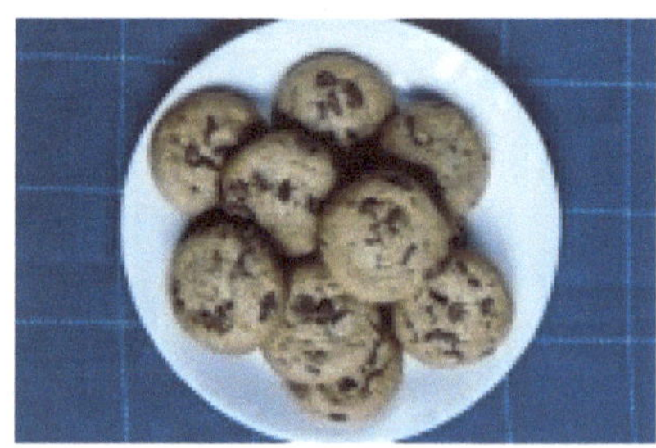

Meringue

Preparation time: 15 minutes
Ingredients:

4 Egg whites
Pinch salt
1/2 Cup Splenda or powdered stevia
1/2 Teaspoon vanilla
1/4 Teaspoon cream of tartar

Instructions:

Heat oven to 400 degrees. Chill metal bowl and beaters. Add egg whites, salt and cream of tartar. Beat on high until they turn white and form stiff peaks. Fold sweetener and vanilla gently into egg whites. Pour atop dessert of choice (pic, etc.). Place in hot oven 5-10 minutes until peaks start browning. Remove. Refrigerate until served.

Mousse 'Cupcakes'

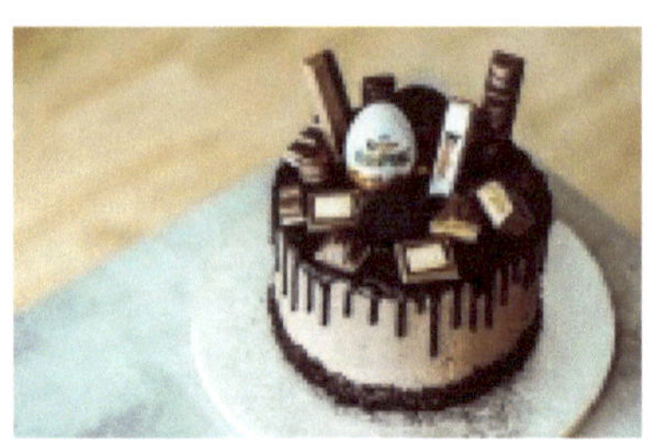

Preparation time: 10 minutes
Ingredients:

- 12 Oz. berries
- 1/3 Cup Splenda or powdered stevia
- 1 Pint heavy whipping cream
- 6 Foil lined cupcake liners

Instructions:

Chill beaters and metal bow. Whip cream with sweetener until peaks form. Add berries and whip. Pour into cupcake liners. If desired, top mousse with crushed nuts or a sprig of mint. Serve immediately. Keep refrigerated.

Variation: Instead of berries, add 2 oz. melted and slightly cooled dark unsweetened baker's chocolate, 1/4 cup unsweetened cocoa.

Ice Cream

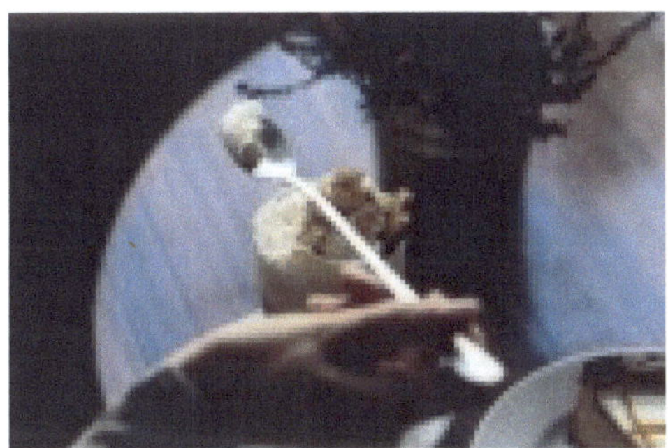

Preparation time: 10 minutes

Ingredients:

- 1 Cup frozen berries of choice
- 2 Tablespoons heavy whipping cream or
  1 canned coconut milk
- 1 Teaspoon vanilla
- 1 Tablespoon Splenda or powdered stevia

Instructions:

With chilled beaters and in a chilled metal bowl, blend heavy cream or milk with vanilla and Splenda until it peaks. Blend in frozen berries. Serve immediately.

Variation: Instead of frozen berries, add 2 oz. dark unsweetened baker's chocolate, melted and slightly cooled or 1/4 cup unsweetened cocoa to create chocolate ice cream. You can also make chocolate banana ice cream by blending in frozen chunks of a banana to the mix, or leave out the chocolate and only use the banana instead of berries. Beware of the carb count in bananas, however, so you don't move yourself out of ketosis.

Chocolate Fudge

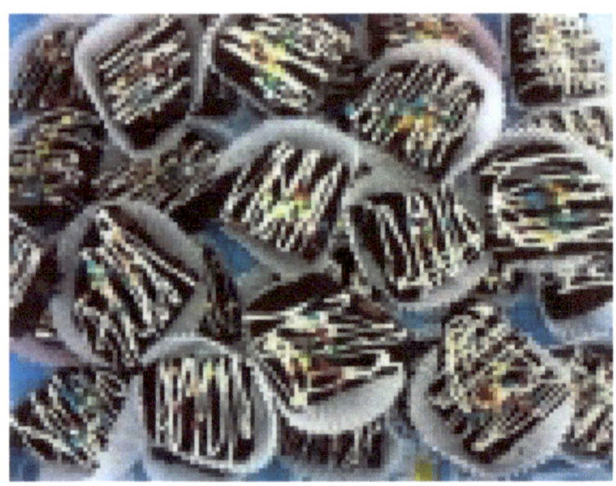

Preparation time: 10 minutes

Ingredients:

2 Oz. dark unsweetened baker's chocolate, melted or
  1/4 Cup unsweetened cocoa
Dash salt
¾ Cup Splenda or powdered stevia
1 Stick unsweetened butter, softened
8 Oz. cream cheese, softened
1 Teaspoon vanilla

Instructions:

Whip butter, cream cheese, sweetener and salt. When creamy, add melted chocolate or cocoa powder. Whip until combined. Pour into a parchment paper lined pan and chill until firm. Lift from pan by paper. Using a wet knife or unflavoured dental floss, slice into serving sized pieces. Serve. Store sealed and refrigerated.

For a variation, add 2 Tablespoons peanut butter. You can also include chopped nuts of your choice in the mix or pressed into the top.

CHAPTER 4
Yummy Drinks

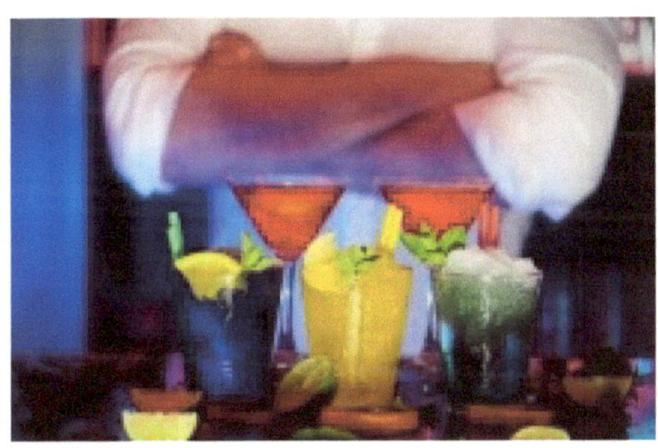

Keto-Friendly Drinks

During a Ketogenic Diet, high-carb drinks, like high-carb foods, must be avoided. A wide variety of beverages, including juice, beer, ice-cream, tea and coffee, contain sugar. Sugary beverages have been linked to a variety of medical conditions, from obesity to an increased risk of diabetes.

Fortunately, the Keto Diet offers many delicious, sugar-free options. Choices for Keto-Friendly Beverages include:

Water: Water is the most suitable choice for hydration and should be taken all day long. Drink at least eight glasses of water per day. To add extra flavor to your water, try fresh mint and lemon peels.

Sparkling water: Sparkling water can make an excellent substitute for soda.

Coffee: Add heavy cream to your coffee for extra benefits.

Green tea: Green tea is delicious and offers many health benefits.

Certain Alcohols: Alcohol should be limited; however, it is perfectly safe to drink low-carb beverages such as vodka, gin or tequila combined with soda water or low-carb beer.

While the following drink recipes focus mainly on non-alcoholic delights, feel free to add white wine, vodka, gin or tequila to them if you prefer something stronger.

Chocolate Milk Shake

Preparation time: 5 minutes
Ingredients:

1 Cup heavy whipping cream
1 Teaspoon vanilla
1 Tablespoon cocoa
1 Tablespoon coconut (optional)
1 Teaspoon butter
1 Teaspoon MCT oil
1 Scoop collagen powder
1 Cup ice
1 Frozen ripe banana (optional)

Instructions:

Blend together and enjoy.

This shake is versatile and ingredients can be swapped out as you wish to make it into your unique desired flavour. Swap out the cocoa for more vanilla and a teaspoon of pineapple flavouring for a **Pina Colada Shake**. Add a tablespoon of nut butter for a **Peanut Butter Cup Shake**. Add a handful of blueberries or strawberries.

Variation: If you're looking for a tasty alcoholic treat, and your diet is at a point where you're comfortable indulging, add a shot glass of white rum. Yum!

Mix it up, and it never gets boring.

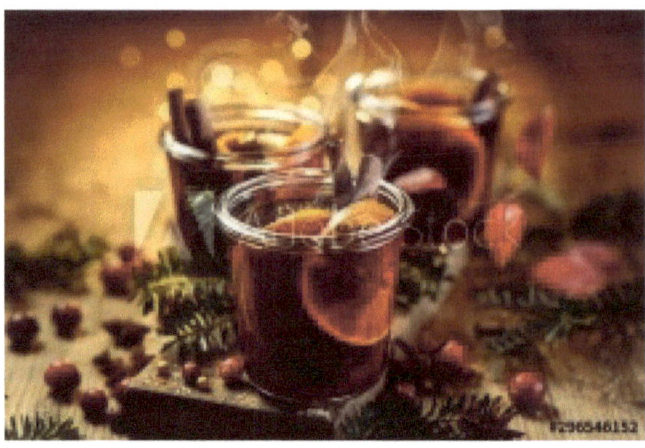

Berry Spritzer

Preparation time: 5 minutes
Ingredients:

½ Cup berry of choice or combination of berries
1/3 Cup powdered stevia or ¼ Cup of agave
½ Cup water
4 Cups white wine

Instructions:

In saucepan, mash berries. Add sweetener and water. On low heat simmer 5 minutes, stirring. Pour wine into mixture and stir to dissolve. Cool in refrigerator for at least an hour or serve in tall glass over ice cubes.

Variation: Fill a glass with ice and a shot of vodka, tequila or white rum. Add berry mixture to fill glass

ABOUT THE AUTHOR

Lyndi Kae brings you benefit of over thirty-six years' research and study of the diet and cooking industry. As with any diet program, Lyndi recommends you consult your physician before beginning.

Enjoy and be sure to check out the other books in the series. See **Also By Lyndi Kae** section in this book.

ALSO BY LYNDI KAE

How To Keto Diet
Simple Keto Cooking
Keto Decadent Desserts
Keto Cheat Sheet
Keto Journal
Keto Shopping Guide
Keto Weekly Meal Planner

CONTACT INFORMATION

Get your copy of **Lyndi Kae's** *Easy Keto Diet,*
Easy Keto Desserts, and other items in the bundle.
See **Also By Lyndi Kae** section of this book for a complete listing.

Reach out to **Lyndi Kae** or follow her Blog at: https://www.HOW-TO-KETO.COM or www.LYNDIKAE,AUTHOR@GMAIL.COM